AMERICAN MEDICAL ASSOCIATION

POCKET GUIDE TO
BACK PAIN

AMERICAN MEDICAL ASSOCIATION

POCKET GUIDE TO

BACK PAIN

RANDOM HOUSE
NEW YORK

LIBRARY OF CONGRESS CATALOGING-IN-PUBLICATION DATA

American Medical Association pocket guide to back pain.
    p. cm.
  Includes index.
  ISBN 0-679-75560-8
  1. Backache—Popular works. 2. Back—Care and hygiene.
I. American Medical Association.
RD771.B217A42 1995
617.5'64—dc20   94-28067

Manufactured in the United States of America

9 8 7 6 5 4 3 2

First Edition

Discounts for bulk purchases are available for sales promo-
tion and premium use. Special editions, including corporate
imprints, can be produced in large quantities. For more information write to Special Markets, Random House, Inc., 201
East 50th Street, New York, NY 10022.

THE AMERICAN MEDICAL ASSOCIATION

James S. Todd, MD — *Executive Vice President*
James F. Rappel — *Group Vice President*
Larry Jellen — *Vice President, Marketing*
Heidi Hough — *Publisher, Consumer Publishing*

Editorial Staff

Patricia Dragisic — *Managing Editor*
Mark Ingebretsen — *Senior Editor*
Daniel Knight — *Editor*
Barbara Scotese — *Editor*
Lisa Riolo — *Editorial Assistant*
Debra Smith — *Editorial Assistant*

Medical Consultants

Roger L. Benson, MD — *Medical Editor*
Srdjan Mirkovic, MD — *Orthopedic Surgery*
Patrick Wempe, PT — *Physical Therapy*
Robert J. Kelsey, Jr., MD — *Obstetrics and Gynecology*

Acknowledgments

Ann Kepler — *Manuscript*
Larry Frederick — *Illustrator*

American Medical Association
Physicians dedicated to the health of America

PREFACE

Back pain is a major health problem, causing aches, discomfort, and distress to many people. In the workplace, back pain is a major cause of absence due to illness.

We have produced the *American Medical Association Pocket Guide to Back Pain* to provide an easy-to-use, reliable source of information on this widespread problem. The book outlines the structure and functioning of your back, discusses the causes of back pain, offers tips on preventing back pain, and reviews the many treatments available—including medication and surgery. The convenient size of this book makes it easy to carry and review anywhere.

If you already have back pain, we as physicians encourage you to take an active part in your treatment by becoming well informed and knowledgeable about it. If you do not have back problems, we encourage you to take steps now to prevent them. This book can help in meeting both goals.

We wish you and your family a healthy, pain-free future.

James S. Todd, MD
Executive Vice President
American Medical Association

CONTENTS

INTRODUCTION

This book—a back owner's manual—offers you information on how to keep your back strong and healthy. Learning about your back—understanding the roles of stress management, exercise, and other factors such as good lifting techniques—is the first step in becoming a partner with your physician in taking care of it.

A healthy back enables you to perform everyday activities with ease, including moving, exercising, working, and even sleeping. Without your back, you could not stand upright, walk, run, lift, bend, reach, dance, or extend your arms in an embrace.

Back pain is common, however, affecting about 80 percent of adults at one time or another in their lives. It is one of the most frequent reasons for a visit to a physician. Back pain causes prolonged discomfort and inconvenience; it also contributes to time lost from work as well as to medical costs and workers' compensation payments.

Back pain can result from a number of causes. Many jobs place significant stress on back muscles. Physical labor performed incorrectly can strain the back. Sitting in a cramped position in front of a computer terminal for long periods of time can also strain the back. Poor posture, lack of exercise, being overweight—to name a few factors—can cause back pain. In addition, disease and injury can lead to chronic back problems.

The normal aging process is also a culprit. As your body grows older, joints and bones change. The discs in your spine are made up of elastic tissue that cushions the friction and permits motion between the bones in the spinal column. With age, the discs lose some flexibility. Many people in their late 40s and 50s put on extra weight; this places extra stress on the bones, joints, and discs, accelerating the effects of the aging process. And people who don't exercise are doing their backs a disservice. Your chances of injury are increased by loss of abdominal muscle tone, poor posture, and using your back improperly (for example, lifting an object in a way that puts too much stress on back bones and muscles; see p.27).

What can you do?

Is there anything you can do about back problems? Yes. Treatments are available for many back problems, and this book will summarize some of the key therapies. In addition, the book will offer tips on how you can help prevent back pain. You will also learn about the structure and function of your back, because understanding how your back is built and how it works is the first step in learning how to take care of it.

You will learn about muscle aches and pains, which are common back problems. In addition, you will learn about back diseases, disorders, and injuries so that you can recognize symptoms that indicate more than just a strained muscle. Knowing when to call your physician is essential to the care of your back.

YOUR BACK— AN OWNER'S MANUAL

Anatomy of the back

The back is a wonderfully interconnected apparatus of bone, muscle, nerve, and ligament. The parts of the back are the spine, made up of the vertebrae; the nerves that run through the vertebrae; the discs of tissue in between the vertebrae; and the ligaments and muscles that support the spine.

The spine

The spine is a structural wonder. A skeletal column formed by 33 bones called vertebrae, the spine supports the body's weight. It also allows movement of the body and helps maintain erect posture with the aid of the muscles and ligaments in the back and abdomen. Finally, the bony spine encloses and protects the spinal cord, the sheath of nerves running directly from the brain down the back (see p.5).

From behind, the vertebrae in a healthy spine form a straight line from the base of your skull to your coccyx, or tailbone. From the side, however, the spinal column forms a naturally S-shaped curve, which is made up of five different regions that help support the weight of your body. The five areas, beginning at the top, are called the cervical (neck), thoracic (chest), and lumbar (lower back) regions, the sacrum, and the coccyx.

More than 100 separate joints connect the bones of the spine to each other and to other bones. Seventy-six facet joints (see p.6) attach the vertebrae to each other, 24 joints connect the thoracic vertebrae to the ribs, two joints connect the sacrum to the hips (called the ilia; hence the term "sacroiliac joint"), and one joint attaches the spine to the skull.

Vertebrae

The seven cervical (neck) vertebrae support the weight of the head and are the smallest and most delicate. The 12 thoracic (chest) vertebrae are larger because they support the additional weight of the shoulders, arms, and ribs. The five lumbar (lower back) vertebrae are the largest of the mobile vertebrae since they carry the greatest weight, which is why this region is most susceptible to pain and disorders. Below the lumbar region, the sacrum and coccyx (tailbone) vertebrae form the immobile base of the spine. In these two areas, the vertebrae fuse together during the growing years of life.

The mobile vertebrae, although varying in size, are relatively similar in structure. Each vertebra has two basic parts: the front (anterior), closest to the front of the body, and the back (posterior), closest to the back of the body. There is also an opening for the spinal cord and seven projections (called processes) for joints and muscle attachments.

The front section is shaped like a drum. The top of each drum is attached to the bottom of the disc above it, and the bottom of each drum adheres to the top of the disc below it. This arrangement creates a vertebrae "sandwich," with the disc as the filling. The drum-shaped section of the vertebra is the weight-bearing part of your back. In fact, some of the larger vertebrae in the lumbar region can support up to several hundred pounds per square inch.

YOUR BACK AND SPINE

More than 100 individual joints connect the bones of the spine (at right) to each other and to other bones. From the side, the natural S-shaped curve of the spine is easy to see. The spine is divided into five areas: cervical (neck), thoracic (chest), lumbar (lower back), sacrum, and coccyx (tailbone).

YOUR BACK AND SPINE

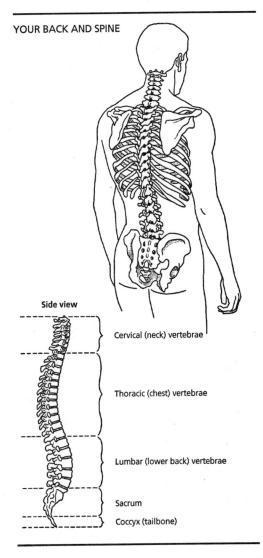

Side view

Cervical (neck) vertebrae

Thoracic (chest) vertebrae

Lumbar (lower back) vertebrae

Sacrum

Coccyx (tailbone)

The rear section of each vertebra contains a hole that forms the spinal canal, which encases the spinal cord. Behind this area seven projections emerge. Four of the projections form joints with other vertebrae. The two projections at the top of the vertebra join with the two projections at the bottom of the vertebra above, forming what are called facet joints that allow you to move and bend your upper body (see p.7).

Two other projections, called transverse processes, emerge from each side of the vertebra, and the last projection, called the spinous process, points toward the rear, behind you, in a downward slant. The muscles of your back are attached to these projections, which act as levers to bend the spine as the muscles contract and relax. The spinous processes are what you feel when you run your fingers up and down your spine.

Although most of the mobile vertebrae are fairly similar in form and function, the first two vertebrae at the top of the spinal column both look and work differently from the others.

The first vertebra has a large central opening with a flat surface on either side to support the skull. It is called the atlas after the mythical Greek giant who carries the earth on his shoulders.

The second vertebra, called the axis, has a post pointing upward at its front that fits into the hole in the atlas. When you shake your head, you are rotating the atlas around the post on the axis. When you nod, you are rocking the skull on the atlas.

Like all bones, vertebrae consist of living tissue. Not only do they provide structure and form for our bodies, they also produce blood cells within their inner core, and act as a storehouse for calcium, phosphorus, and other minerals, moving them in and out of the bloodstream according to the body's needs.

Discs

Between each two vertebrae is a pad of elastic cartilage tissue called a disc (short for intervertebral disc). Acting as shock absorbers and cushions between the bones, discs have tough, fibrous outer regions and soft centers. Because the soft center is mostly water, it is very elastic and can change its shape and then return to its original form, which gives the spine flexibility (see p.14). For example, when gravity exerts its force on your upright body, your discs are shortened as water leaves their centers and is absorbed into the bloodstream. When you are in bed, without the pressure of gravity on your erect spine, discs absorb water from the blood. The result is that you may be an inch or two taller in the morning than you are at the end of the day.

TWO VERTEBRAE

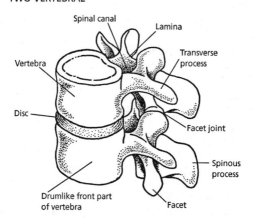

Vertebrae, the basic unit of the spine, are interconnected by joints, ligaments, and muscles. Discs of elastic cartilage tissue between the vertebrae allow flexibility.

As you age, your discs dry out; they lose the ability to absorb fluid, and the amount of fluid they contain slowly decreases, making them less flexible.

Nerves

Each vertebra has an opening behind its body to allow the spinal cord to run through it. These holes line up to form the spinal canal through which the spinal cord runs from the base of the brain to a point located a few inches above the waist. Below this point, individual nerve fibers continue down the canal in strands that resemble a horse's tail, and that is why they are called the cauda equina, Latin for "horse's tail."

Whenever the brain sends out a command to or receives a message from another part of the body, the information is transmitted in the form of an electro-chemical signal along the nerve fibers in the spinal cord. The spinal cord branches along its length, sending off on either side smaller nerve bundles, called nerve roots, from between each two vertebrae. In turn, these nerves combine and rebranch until they have developed a complete network of nerves for the entire body.

Each pair of nerve roots (one on each side) serves a different part of the body. For example, nerves emerging from between some of the cervical (neck) vertebrae send signals to muscles that move the shoulders, wrists, and fingers. Nerves originating from between lumbar (lower back) vertebrae send signals to muscles in the hips and knees. Some of the nerves exiting from the lumbar region join nerves emerging through holes in the sacrum to form a single, large nerve, called the sciatic nerve (from Latin for "hip"), one on either side of the body. Back problems that affect the roots of the sciatic nerve can cause sciatica (see p.61), a particular type of pain that often travels down the back of the leg.

SPINAL NERVES

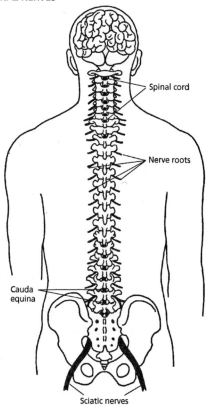

Spinal cord

Nerve roots

Cauda equina

Sciatic nerves

Messages to and from the brain are carried along the spinal cord (shown from the rear). The nerve roots branch off and carry messages to various areas of the body. A few inches above the waist, the spinal cord divides into individual nerve fibers, the cauda equina ("horse's tail"). The two sciatic nerves run down both sides of the body.

It is easy to see that the unique position of the spinal cord means that back problems can have far-reaching or long-range effects on the normal functioning of the nervous system. Any diseased or irritated bone, disc, or other part of the spine (such as ligaments) can press on the spinal cord, a nerve root, or both, leading to discomfort and symptoms in your back or along a nerve heading toward another part of the body.

Ligaments

Ligaments are tough bands of connective tissue that connect one bone to another. Because of these connections, ligaments control much of the movement in your joints.

In your back, ligaments support the spine and also help prevent excessive movements that may cause damage or pain; for example, a ligament can prevent you from moving a joint beyond its normal range. Several ligaments provide support for the joints of the mobile vertebrae, and others support the discs and vertebral bones.

There are two long ligaments. One, the anterior longitudinal ligament, travels as one long band over the vertebrae and discs in the front of the spine throughout its length. The second, the posterior longitudinal ligament, also runs as a single band over the rear of the vertebrae and discs to strengthen the disc joints. Other short ligaments tie together the projections at the rear of the vertebrae.

Muscles

The back has many different kinds of muscles. Short muscles support the spine and allow you to make delicate movements. As the muscles attached to projections on the vertebrae expand and contract, they pull and release the projections like levers, enabling the back to bend and rotate within the limits set by the ligaments.

The short muscles attached to the facet joints also maneuver the facet joints like levers. However, the construction of each joint defines its ability to move forward, backward, or sideways.

Covering the short muscles are many layers of longer back muscles. Medium-length muscles stretch from one vertebra to another several inches away. Over the medium-length muscles lies a group of muscles that runs the entire length of the spine; these are called the erector spinae, Latin for "erector of the spine."

The erector spinae is one of the most important supports and manipulators of the spine. When it is contracted, the erector spinae bends the spine backward. When only one side is contracted, the spine bends sideways. And it braces the spine from the rear so that you do not topple forward.

Yet another layer of muscles covers the erector spinae group. While these muscles are attached to the vertebrae, they do not directly support or move the spine. Rather, they move some other part of the body. Those in the upper back move the shoulders and arms. Large muscles in the chest area move the ribs to enable you to breathe. And the lower back has muscles attached to the hips that move your legs.

In contrast to the layers of muscles at the back of the spine, there are very few muscles in front of the spine, except for the neck area. Therefore, the work of moving the spine forward is the responsibility of the muscles that make up the abdominal wall. There are several layers of abdominal muscles, and when all of them are contracted, the spine bends forward. If the abdominal muscles are contracted on one side, the spine moves sideways.

BACK MUSCLES

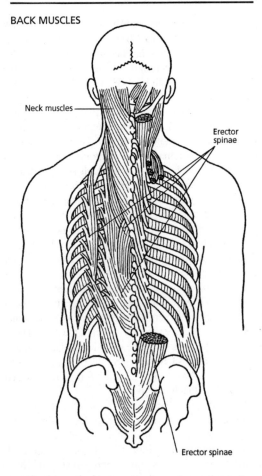

Neck muscles

Erector spinae

Erector spinae

Different types and layers of back muscles work together to help the back move freely. The erector spinae group of muscles helps to support and move the spine.

Supporting the spinal column from the front in the chest region is the job performed by the ribs. Attached to the vertebrae in the back, the ribs curve into a cage and fasten to the breastbone in front. Lower down, the lumbar (lower back) region of the spine depends on the abdominal muscles to brace it in front. The normal tension in these muscles prevents the spine from falling backward.

How the back works

A healthy back synchronizes all of its parts to move in a coordinated, fluid manner. The key to this smooth motion is that the spine's many individual vertebrae are able to move and bend because of the elasticity of the discs between them. Coupled with strong muscles and ligaments that limit damaging movements, the back is able to use four basic motions—bending forward, bending backward, bending sideways, and rotating—to perform daily tasks with ease.

Although the individual joints between vertebrae do not have a wide range of movement, collectively they provide the spine with a great range of flexibility. The key component is the disc between each two vertebrae. The discs are so elastic that they can change their shape to accommodate movement.

If the back bends to the left or right, the discs will expand and stretch on the outside of the bend while simultaneously compressing and bulging on the inside of the bend. This allows the vertebrae to move in relation to each other.

Thanks to the support of the abdominal muscles, the back bends forward most easily. Back muscles, however, also allow you to stand erect, bend backward to look at the sky, lean to the side, or rotate your head to look over your shoulder.

SPINE FLEXIBILITY

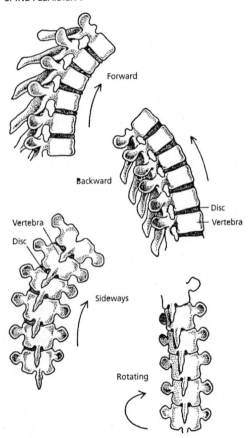

The spine is flexible and can move forward or backward, bend to the side, and twist (rotate). The elastic discs between the vertebrae make possible this wide range of movements.

Just how flexible is the spine? The neck region is the most flexible. Its muscles and discs allow you to move your neck in all directions. In contrast, the chest area is encased in the rib cage, which prevents that part of the spine from bending very far forward. In addition, the projections on the back of the vertebrae in this region overlap closely, so it is more difficult for them to bend backward.

Below the rib cage, the large vertebrae of the lumbar (lower back) region permit you to bend your lower back forward and backward with little trouble, but they limit your ability to twist. And the sacrum—the large, wedge-shaped bone near the bottom of the spine—is the least flexible. Not only are its vertebrae fused together, but it is attached to the pelvic bones and really moves only when the pelvis moves.

The spine and back provide a sound structure to support our upright posture. Nevertheless, because of the load we place on our backs every day, especially on the lower spine, back pain, disorders, and diseases can occur. Given the many interlinking parts of the back, it is not surprising that some occasionally malfunction, leading to pain, discomfort, and loss of normal motion. When that happens, we realize that we cannot take the health of our backs for granted. It's important to think about preventive care for our backs.

TAKING CARE OF YOUR BACK

Preventive back care

It's not always possible to prevent back pain, but in many cases establishing good health habits can forestall back problems. Furthermore, once you have experienced back pain, you will want to learn how to avoid a repeat episode. A good preventive regimen can help prevent pain from occurring again.

Back basics

There are some fundamental steps you can take to promote the well-being of your back.

Controlling your weight

A balanced, nutritious diet contributes to the overall health of your body, including your back. In addition, a healthy diet can also help you maintain your ideal weight and stay trim.

Being overweight can put excess pressure on your back; the strain of only a few extra pounds on the lower back can lead to problems. Often, extra weight accumulates in the abdominal area, especially for men, creating a potbelly. The bigger the potbelly, the greater the strain on the back, because extra weight in front tends to pull the body forward. To compensate for this, the back muscles must tense, thus increasing the potential for problems and pain in the lower back.

Losing weight is not easy, and it is rarely accomplished by a crash diet or stringent diet. Diets like those may work initially, but often the dieter begins to feel deprived and frustrated. Many people succumb to temptation and give up, often regaining any weight they have lost and even gaining more.

A sensible weight-loss program combines nutritious food choices and exercise (see below). Your diet should provide the appropriate nutrients, but, more importantly, should be one you can live with—for life. Reducing your intake of fats and sweets is a start. Plan your meals to include ample portions of fresh fruits and vegetables, complex carbohydrates such as pasta and whole-grain products, and nonfat or low-fat foods. Consider making meat a side dish in a meal rather than the main dish.

Gradually create a diet that you can live with and enjoy. Your weight loss will be gradual, but you will be more likely to keep the extra pounds off. An added benefit is that you increase the amount of fiber in your meals when you add fresh fruits, vegetables, and whole-grain products. Adequate fiber along with liquids helps prevent constipation, and people who have had back problems know how straining during a bowel movement can trigger back pain.

Exercise

Exercising regularly helps you keep your weight under control, which is beneficial to your back. Exercise also contributes to flexibility and mobility. Following an exercise program is important, but exercise does not have to be arduous. Talk to your physician before starting an exercise program, especially if you have back problems, other health concerns, or if you're over 40 and have not been exercising. If your back problems are serious, your physician may recommend seeking the help of a physical therapist to develop an appropriate exercise program (see p.39). Many people with back problems enjoy swimming because it exercises many muscles in the body while the water supports the spine. It is probably best, however, to avoid the breaststroke, since arching your back may be uncomfortable.

Walking is also an excellent exercise. Walking places less pressure on the lower back than does sitting in a chair that does not support your back. Walking also is free, does not require special equipment (except shoes with adequate cushioning), and can be done at any time or in any place. In bad weather, go to an enclosed shopping mall for a brisk walk. In fact, some shopping malls welcome walking clubs sponsored by local hospitals, health clinics, or senior centers.

Exercise that requires your skeletal system to bear weight is very important to maintaining the health of your bones. Weight-bearing exercise stimulates the body to rebuild old bone with new bone, and is very important in preventing osteoporosis. (See p.31 for specific exercises to prevent back pain.)

Reducing stress

Good nutrition and regular exercise not only contribute to good health but also help combat stress and anxiety. The precise relationship between stress and back pain is not known. But many people with back problems have noticed a link between stress and pain. If you are unusually apprehensive or tense, especially over long periods of time, you may be experiencing the type of stress that can bring about or aggravate illness, including back pain.

No matter what your worries—finances, work problems, health, loss, or large changes in your life—how you handle these stressful factors or situations may affect your health. In time the body's responses to prolonged stress, including tense muscles, rapid heartbeat, and sweating, can translate into ongoing backache, pounding heartbeat, or indigestion. When you begin to experience such symptoms with no apparent physical cause, it is time to make changes in your daily life.

First, try to determine what you are anxious about. It may be helpful to categorize your concerns as problems you can do something about or circumstances over which you have no control. Then take action to relieve the stress that is due to situations you can do something about, and try to stop worrying about situations that you cannot change or control. Here are a few suggestions to improve how you feel about your daily life:

- Talk about your problem. Discuss it with a friend, family member, or trusted mentor. Often simply expressing your concerns brings some relief.

- Exercise regularly. Physical exertion is an uncomplicated and a time-honored stress reducer.

- Eat a well-balanced diet. Remember, too, that alcohol and caffeine (found in coffee, tea, cola, and chocolate) may increase anxiety.

- Plan your day realistically in terms of time and energy needed.

- Get enough rest. You can manage daily stresses better if you are rested and alert.

- Breathe deeply and evenly for 5 minutes when you feel the beginning of tension at work or at home. Or meditate: close your eyes and focus for a few minutes on a pleasant and calming image, or one that has no emotional meaning for you. These exercises can be done anywhere and may help you through a particularly stressful episode.

- Plan a relaxing activity that you enjoy, such as walking, reading, needlework, photography, listening to music, or gardening.

- Volunteer your time and energy. If you have time on your hands or feel lonely or isolated, volunteer to help others. Community groups, churches, and educational organizations are usually looking for additional volunteers.

If you are unable to alleviate your stress after trying some of these suggestions, talk with your physician about any ongoing stress that may be contributing to your back pain.

Preventing osteoporosis

Another source of back pain is a condition called osteoporosis, a loss of bone tissue and weakening of the bones. (Osteoporosis means "porous bones.") Throughout life, your body replaces old bone tissue with new. During childhood, new tissue forms faster than old tissue breaks down. This enables children's bones to grow. At around age 35, however, bone tissue begins to break down faster than it is replaced, and bone loss begins. Eventually, the loss may lead to a condition called osteoporosis (see p.67).

Osteoporosis is diagnosed when the bones have become so fragile and weak that a minor fall or even a vigorous hug can fracture a bone. The bones most commonly affected are the vertebrae, ribs, wrists, or hips. People most often affected are women, particularly in the years after menopause because of lowered levels of the female hormone estrogen, which helps prevent bone loss. Although osteoporosis can affect men, women are more likely to develop it, in part because they have less overall bone matter than men, and therefore lower calcium reserves.

Can you slow the rate of bone loss or even prevent it? Yes. The key is the mineral calcium. Bone is the storehouse for calcium, and it is calcium that keeps your bones firm and strong. If your calcium intake is low, your body takes calcium from your bones to compensate, leading to loss of bone density.

How much calcium do you need each day? The recommended dietary allowance for adults 25 and older is 800 milligrams (mg) per day, although many experts believe that 1,000 mg is needed. Adolescents and young adults 11 to 24 need 1,200 mg to 1,500 mg every day, as do women who are pregnant or breast-feeding. Studies have shown that the average calcium intake for middle-aged and older women is between 400 and 550 mg per day. This is one reason why osteoporosis is more prevalent among older women. Women past menopause should get 1,000 mg to 1,500 mg of calcium every day; women over 65 should get 1,500 mg per day.

The best source of calcium is milk or milk products. To reduce saturated fat intake, choose low-fat or nonfat milk. One cup of milk contains approximately 300 mg of calcium. If you are unable to digest milk easily, ask your physician about commercial products that replace the missing enzyme lactase that your body needs to digest milk.

Other good sources of calcium are calcium-fortified orange juice, broccoli, dark green vegetables, canned salmon and sardines (including the bones), and tofu. Vitamin D is also necessary for calcium absorption. Although vitamin D is not present in many common foods, your body manufactures most of the vitamin D it needs when you are exposed to sunlight. In addition, most brands of milk are fortified with vitamin D.

Along with diet, weight-bearing exercise, in which bones work against muscles or gravity, helps increase bone density and slow bone loss. Exercise does not have to be complicated and difficult to fit into your schedule. Walking, dancing, and running are good

21

exercises; swimming is not helpful in preventing osteo-porosis, because your bones do not bear weight in water. Walk on your lunch hour three or more times per week. Run in place for at least 5 minutes four or five times per week. Climb stairs rather than use the elevator. Get off the bus several blocks from your des-tination and walk the rest of the way. Walk when you run errands, or at least park your car at the far end of a parking lot. Every bit of exercise helps.

Hormone replacement therapy can also minimize the risk of osteoporosis in women after menopause. Women reaching menopause should not wait for prob-lems to occur; hormone replacement therapy is most beneficial when given early. Discuss the potential benefits and drawbacks of hormone replacement ther-apy with your physician.

Preventing injury

Maintaining good posture

Preventing injury to your back begins with learning good posture. Each person has a natural posture depend-ing on build, health, and age. For a healthy posture, you should stand comfortably without exaggerating any of the spine's curves and with your head, torso, and legs balanced in alignment.

One posture that seems to contribute to backaches is the one that you may have been taught is "good" posture, that is, the "attention" posture: shoulders back, chest up, stomach flat, and buttocks protruding. This stance exaggerates the arch of the lower back, caus-ing the posture called swayback. Swayback also results when you stand with slumping shoulders, a sagging lower back, or a protruding abdomen. People who are overweight or women who are pregnant often arch their backs to compensate for extra weight in the front.

When a swayback posture arches the spine backward, the discs naturally bulge backward also to permit the motion. People who have weakened or diseased discs may feel pain if the bulging disc presses on a nearby nerve. Swayback may also intensify the pain of arthritis or other diseases of the spinal joints by applying pressure on the affected joints.

POSTURE AND THE SPINE

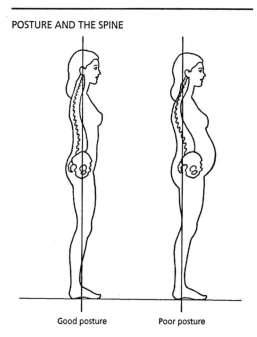

Good posture   Poor posture

For good posture, your body's weight should be well balanced; your head, spine, hips, and legs should be centered (see left). In poor posture, your weight is shifted forward (for instance, by pregnancy; see right), causing you to arch your back; your body is no longer centered and in alignment.

To test your posture, stand with your back against a doorframe, lightly pressing your upper back, buttocks, and heels to the frame. Slip your hand in the space between the doorframe and the small of your back. Your hand should slide in easily and touch both the doorframe and your back. If there is extra space between your back and the frame, you may be arching your back too much.

If that is the case, the standing pelvic tilt exercise may help you correct the excessive arch. Remove your hand, and move your feet a few inches away from the doorframe. Flatten your back against the frame without bending your knees or hips. This will force you to tilt your pelvis so that the lower part moves away from the doorframe and the upper part rolls toward it. This pelvic tilt flattens out the spine and helps increase its flexibility. Repeating this exercise can also relieve back pain caused by an unnatural arch in the lower back.

Standing

When you need to stand for long periods of time, stand with one foot resting on a small stool, step, or chair rung. This bends both hip and knee, flattening any excessive arch in your back and relaxing muscles that contribute to arching of the spine. This position also releases any pressure on the sciatic nerve, which can be a source of pain. Try to adopt this position whenever you must stand at a work counter, workbench, drawing board, ironing board, or anywhere else for any length of time.

Sitting

Contrary to a widespread belief that sitting rests your back, sitting actually increases the load on your lower back, particularly if your back is unsupported. Sitting shifts the weight of the upper body forward, forcing

TESTING YOUR POSTURE

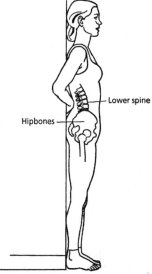

Lower spine

Hipbones

Standing with your back against a doorframe, slip your hand in the space between the doorframe and the small of your back. Your hand should slide in easily and touch both doorframe and back. If it doesn't, remove your hand, and move your feet a few inches from the door-frame. Tilt your pelvis by flattening your back against the doorframe, but don't bend your knees and hips.

the back muscles to work harder to prevent you from toppling forward.

A common cause of back pain is a prolapsed disc (see p.54), a condition in which disc material protrudes out of the disc and presses against a nerve. Although a prolapsed disc is often caused by strenuous activity, people who sit for long periods of time may also develop the condition.

HOW TO SELECT A COMFORTABLE CHAIR

- Be sure the chair is adjustable so that you can adapt it to fit your body.
- Select a back support that fits your back; you may want it slanted backward or curved to conform to the natural arch of your back.
- Choose a chair with armrests; resting your arms helps decrease the load on your back.
- Look for a seat height that allows you to place your feet flat on the floor with knees bent at a right angle.
- Make sure the seat depth is not too deep (that is, does not force you to sit with your back rounded or sit forward without resting against the back support) or too shallow (that is, it cuts into the backs of your thighs).
- Select a chair that accommodates the height of your desk. Or, conversely, select a desk that works with your chair.

Remember that although you may spend much of your time in your office chair, you also spend time in your car. Use the same criteria in selecting or adjusting car seats that you use in selecting chairs.

If you have a desk job that requires long intervals of sitting, what can you do to alleviate the stress placed on your back? Some people work at standup desks. Others take and make all telephone calls while standing up. Still others try to find opportunities to get up and walk at regular intervals.

Investing in a well-designed, well-made chair can also reduce the stress of sitting. The main criterion in selecting a chair is your individual comfort; a chair may be suitable for a colleague but uncomfortable for you. Your best bet is to shop until you find a chair that meets your needs. If you need to work with a chair selected by your employer, be sure to adjust the back and the seat to help the chair support your back. (See How to select a comfortable chair, this page.)

Bending

Bending places more stress on the back than sitting. When you bend forward, you force the erector spinae muscles in the back to tense in order to counteract the tendency to fall forward.

One way to protect your back while gardening or picking up something from the floor is to squat or work on your hands and knees rather than to bend over with your legs straight. Proper tools also help. Lightweight tools with long handles—rakes, brooms, and vacuum cleaners—allow you to work without bending and straining your back.

Another safeguard for deskbound workers is adjusting the height of work surfaces, if possible, so that they are not too low in relation to the height of the seat. This is especially important for people who sit on a stool and do close work at a drawing board.

Lifting

Two situations increase the risk of back strain when you are lifting an object: one is bending from the waist and the other is holding a load far out in front of you.

When you bend from the waist to lift a heavy load, you are adding the weight of your body to the load, and you are depending on the delicate back muscles to do all the work. Likewise, holding a load out in front of you forces the back to work harder, generating more pressure on your lower back.

Following the simple rules listed under The correct way to lift, on the next page, will minimize the strain on your back that lifting can cause. However, if you already have back problems, ask your physician about how much you can safely lift, especially if lifting is involved in your job.

THE CORRECT WAY TO LIFT
Here are some guidelines to help keep your back healthy when you need to lift something heavy:

- Place your feet firmly with one foot slightly ahead of the other for stability.
- Bend your knees, not your waist. Keep your back as close to vertical as possible.
- Use your abdominal muscles to support your spine when you lift. Tighten your abdominal muscles as soon as you grasp the object.
- Lift with your leg muscles. Using your powerful leg muscles to bear the weight of the load helps prevent strain on the weaker back muscles.
- Do not twist your torso. Rotating your body while lifting a heavy load adds to the risk of injury.
- Hold the load close to your body. When lifting something from the inside of a container or your car trunk, place one foot on the edge of the container or bumper of the car to get the leverage you need to lift the object close to your body.

Sleeping

Many people with back problems find that sleeping on their sides with hips and knees bent is the most comfortable position. If you prefer sleeping on your back, you can achieve the same comfort if you place a pillow under your knees to support them and prevent muscle fatigue in your legs. This bending of the hips and knees flattens the arch of the spine and relieves tension that can cause back problems.

If you have back problems, sleeping on your stomach may be uncomfortable. Lying facedown exaggerates the natural arch in your lower back and can lead to a backache.

THE CORRECT WAY TO LIFT

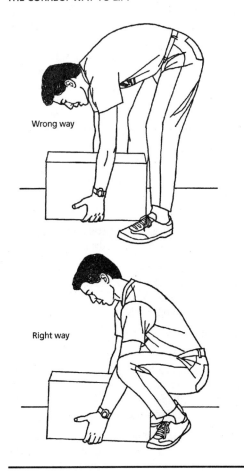

Wrong way

Right way

What about beds? Like selecting a chair, choosing a bed depends on your own comfort and individual needs. Some people are more comfortable with a hard mattress or a mattress supported by a hard board. Others prefer waterbeds or even reclining chairs. Few people like a soft mattress. A disadvantage of a soft mattress is its tendency to allow the spine to sag, which can irritate the back muscles. Shop around and select a bed that is most comfortable for you; don't be shy about lying on a bed at the store, to make sure that it's right for you.

Other preventive steps

Here are a few more tips to prevent back problems:

- Don't cradle the telephone between your neck and shoulder; this can lead to neck and shoulder pain. Invest in a lightweight headset or receiver cushion if you spend a lot of time on the phone.

- Don't hold a book or newspaper too close or too far away, as this can strain back muscles. If you are having trouble seeing print on the page, have your vision checked by an ophthalmologist.

- When driving long distances, stop every hour or so to walk around.

- Balance shoulder bags, briefcases, and gear carriers on both shoulders. If heavy loads cannot be evenly distributed, shift them from side to side as you walk to prevent backaches.

- Avoid wearing high-heeled shoes. High heels tilt the lower back forward, placing pressure on joints, muscles, and ligaments in the lower back.

- Don't use foam rubber pillows; they are a prime cause of neck stiffness. Instead, choose pillows made of feathers, down, or manufactured fibers.

Back conditioning exercises

In addition to maintaining a regular exercise program, you can also perform specific flexibility and strengthening exercises to help prevent injury or reinjury to your back. Before doing any of these exercises, however, ask your physician what kind of exercise is best for your condition.

The most beneficial exercises help strengthen the lumbar (lower back) muscles and the abdominal support muscles, thereby helping to stabilize the spine. These exercises help your muscles maintain a comfortably upright posture, which will relieve most back pain. Do these exercises on a firm surface. Rest a few moments between each exercise. Remember that these exercises should never increase your back pain or leg symptoms. If they do, stop exercising promptly and consult your physician.

Abdominal exercises

Repeat each of the following exercises 12 times.

- Lie on your back with your knees bent, feet flat on the floor, arms at your side. Tighten your abdominal muscles and press them down to flatten your back against the floor. Hold for a count of five.

- Lie on your back with your legs straight out. Raise your head and shoulders off the floor with your arms out straight pointing toward your feet. Only your shoulder blades should leave the ground; do not do a full sit-up. Hold for a count of five.

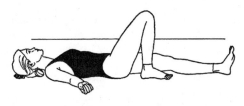

- Lie on your back and tighten your abdominal muscles to flatten your back against the floor. Raise one knee by sliding the foot toward your buttocks, then lower it back down. Repeat with other knee.

Pelvic tilt exercises

Repeat each of the following exercises 12 times (except as noted).

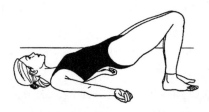

- Lie on your back with your knees bent and your feet flat on the floor. Push your lower back flat against the floor by contracting your stomach muscles and tilting your pelvis forward. Then arch your back away from the floor, keeping your hips and buttocks on the floor. Then raise both back and buttocks off the floor and hold for a count of five.

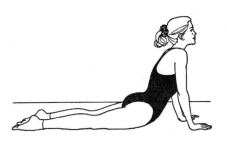

- Lie on your stomach as if you were going to do a push-up, with your hands underneath your shoulders. Press up with your arms while keeping your pelvis on the floor until your arms are straight. Hold for a count of five.

- Lie on your back with your arms at your sides and your legs flat on the floor in front of you. Wrap your arms around one knee and pull it toward your chest. Return to the starting position. Repeat with other knee.

- Lie on your stomach and prop your head and shoulders up on your elbows. Hold for 2 minutes. (Repeat this one 5 times only.)

- Lie on your back with your arms at your sides. Wrap your arms around both knees and pull them to your chest.

Stretching exercises

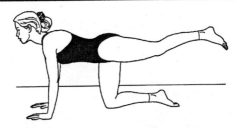

- Get down on your hands and knees, and arch your back upward while tucking your chin toward your chest. Lift the knee of one leg toward your forehead, and then extend that leg straight out behind you while looking up. Try to keep your leg in a straight line with your back; do not lift your leg higher than the level of your back. Repeat with the other leg. Repeat five times.

EXERCISE TIPS
- These exercises are designed to help prevent back pain. If you already have back pain, it's best to speak with your physician before starting these exercises or any others.

- Stretching exercises should be performed with slow and deliberate movements. Abrupt or sudden stretching movements can actually injure your back.

- Do the exercises in a relaxed manner; don't rush through them.

- If exercising increases the pain in your back or legs, stop exercising promptly and talk to your physician.

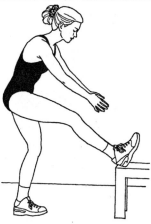

- Hamstring stretch: Stand with your back straight. Place one foot on a stool, keeping that leg straight. Flex your ankle toward you so that your toes are pointed up. Lean forward, reaching your hands toward your feet, to gently stretch the muscles in the back of the thigh. Hold for a count of 20. Repeat with the other leg. Repeat five times.

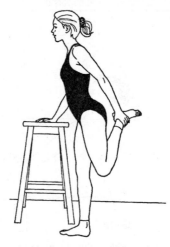

- Quadriceps stretch: Stand on one foot and grasp your other ankle by bending your knee. Hold this position, without leaning forward, for a count of 20. Repeat five times.

When to seek help for back pain

If, despite all your efforts to strengthen your back and prevent problems, you suddenly have pain in your back, what should you do?

Some periods of back pain are ordinary aches that you can attribute to an afternoon of gardening or an evening of bowling. However, certain types of pain signal the need to see your physician either for treatment or to rule out a more serious problem. Seek help if you:

- have a backache that lasts longer than 2 weeks.

- experience pain that shoots down your leg toward your foot or down your arm toward your hand. This kind of pain, with or without a backache, may mean that a prolapsed disc (see p.54) or other tissue is pressing against a nerve. **Warning:** Pain in your arm may mean that you are having a heart attack; seek medical help immediately.

- have numbness in your leg or foot or in your arm or hand. Again, an abnormality such as a prolapsed disc (see p.54) may be pressing on a nerve and interrupting sensations being relayed from your arm or leg to your brain.

- have back pain that wakes you from sleep. Most backaches diminish when you lie down, but if you awaken with pain, there may be an underlying disease that should be diagnosed and treated.

- are unable to control your bladder or bowels. (This symptom occurs only rarely.) An abnormality such as a prolapsed disc may be pressing on critical nerves serving those areas of your body.

Warning: If your back pain begins rapidly and gets worse rapidly and is accompanied by a fever, chills, and/or any of the symptoms listed previously, then you may need immediate medical help. If you cannot contact your physician right away, go to a hospital emergency department.

Finally, if you have any pain or discomfort that worries you, always contact your physician. Prevention is always better than treatment, and if you and your physician can diagnose and treat a back problem early, you are in a good position to prevent more serious trouble later on.

Types of treatment

There are several treatment options for back pain. As with any kind of therapy, some treatments may help you and others may not. The following overview will give you information you can use in discussing treatment choices with your physician.

Bed rest

Going to bed is instinctively the first way most people react to back pain. And, indeed, lying down in the proper position reduces the load on your back. If you injure a limb, you can support it with a sling, crutch, or cane, but lying down is the only way to prevent a sore back from bearing the weight of your body. By lying down to reduce the pressure on your back, you are giving the structures in your back time to heal.

Bed rest may be necessary for a few days or a few weeks, depending on the cause of the back pain and the severity of the condition. Bed rest is often the treatment of choice for such disorders as arthritis, spinal stenosis, injury, or compression fractures (see Other possible spinal conditions, p.62).

Some physicians prescribe complete bed rest in the hospital or at home. In both cases, you are strongly advised not to get out of bed for any reason. As your condition improves, you may be allowed out of bed to use the bathroom, bathe, or eat. Your physician will help you decide how and when to begin to resume your normal routine.

Bed rest is not without undesirable side effects. Lying in bed increases bone loss; its effect is the opposite of that produced by weight-bearing exercise, which helps prevent osteoporosis. In addition, bed rest weakens muscles from lack of use. Talk to your physician about the pros and cons of bed rest. In many cases, getting up and resuming your routine after a few days decreases the length of disability and improves the chance of a good outcome.

If you are a single adult or if you are alone for long hours, getting bed rest may be a challenge for you. Help is available, however. Your physician or your local community health agency may be able to arrange for home health services. These may include nursing, physical therapy, and homemaker services. Medical procedures (such as blood tests), if needed, would be performed by a qualified visiting nurse. If you are confined to bed, a home health aide with nonmedical nursing skills can help you by performing such tasks as changing bed sheets and helping you with personal hygiene. A social worker may be able to help you with the emotional and practical problems of bed rest.

Rehabilitative exercise

After you have gone through a bout of back pain and your problem has been diagnosed (and perhaps after a long period of bed rest), your physician may recommend sessions of rehabilitative exercise. For this treatment, you may be referred to a physical therapist (also called a physiotherapist).

Physical therapists develop exercises to help you overcome pain or stiffness, or to correct problems with posture. In the beginning, a physical therapist may do all the work, moving your limbs (and thereby exercising your joints and muscles) to restore flexibility and muscle tone. Later, as your condition improves, the therapist will guide you through an exercise program that you can do on your own. Physical therapists also use heat to relax muscles in spasm (involuntary tightening), cold to numb pain, massage to loosen muscles, or whirlpool baths to warm and gently massage tense muscles.

When your treatment is complete, the physical therapist can help evaluate your work demands and habits, your lifestyle, and other factors that may affect the health of your back. Working with your physician, your physical therapist may make specific recommendations for preventing back pain and avoiding back injury. Patient education, formal or informal, is usually included as part of physical therapy.

Medication

There are several medications that your physician may recommend to help relieve your back pain. If your physician suggests medication, be sure to mention any other medications you are taking, both prescription and nonprescription. This will help prevent a drug interaction if you are taking drugs prescribed by another physician. Also tell your physician if you are pregnant or could become pregnant.

Ask your physician if you should avoid certain foods, drinks, or activities such as driving while taking a medication. Be certain about the dosage; if you have any questions, ask for clarification. And ask for information about storing the medication so that it remains effective and safe.

Be sure to find out how and when to take the medication. Inquire about possible side effects, both minor and temporary ones and those serious enough to need medical attention. Never leave your physician's office unsure about how to use your medication effectively and safely.

Analgesic drugs

Analgesic drugs are pain relievers. If your back pain is mild to moderate, your physician may suggest acetaminophen or a nonsteroidal anti-inflammatory drug

(NSAID) such as ibuprofen, naproxen, or aspirin. Nonsteroidal anti-inflammatory drugs are so named to distinguish them from corticosteroids, which are more powerful anti-inflammatories but with potentially serious side effects.

All three of these common nonprescription pain relievers work the same way: they inhibit the body's production of hormonelike substances called prostaglandins that trigger fever, pain, and inflammation. Aspirin, ibuprofen, naproxen, and other nonsteroidal anti-inflammatory drugs fight prostaglandins that set off all three symptoms. Acetaminophen works only against those responsible for fever and pain; that is, acetaminophen does not reduce inflammation.

Your physician may also prescribe nonsteroidal anti-inflammatory drugs if the nonprescription remedies do not work. Common prescription nonsteroidal anti-inflammatory medications include fenoprofen, indomethacin, meclofenamate, phenylbutazone, sulindac, and tolmetin.

While all of these analgesic medications can be very effective, it's important to note that they have side effects. For example, nonsteroidal anti-inflammatory drugs can cause stomach upset and impair the blood's ability to clot. Excessive or prolonged use of aspirin can cause intestinal bleeding and ringing in the ears. Acetaminophen has fewer side effects than aspirin, although it can cause skin rash or pain during urination. However, since acetaminophen does not fight inflammation, it is probably not a good choice for back pain.

For severe back pain, your physician may prescribe a narcotic painkiller, such as codeine, hydrocodone, or propoxyphene. These medications work by mimicking the action of the brain's natural pain relievers, called endorphins, which block the transmission of pain signals within the nervous system. These drugs are usually prescribed only for short periods, however, because they are addictive and are not necessary for long-term pain control.

Muscle relaxants and antidepressants

If your back pain is caused by muscle spasms resulting from an injury or arthritis, your physician may prescribe muscle relaxants. These medications work on the central nervous system (brain and spinal cord), blocking nerve cells that transmit signals from the nervous system to the muscles. This reduces muscle contraction and relaxes muscles in spasm. Often these medications are used to allow you to undergo physical therapy. Common muscle relaxants are baclofen, cyclobenzaprine, methocarbamol, and diazepam.

Muscle relaxants can cause drowsiness and may relax all the muscles in the body, not just the sore ones in your back. Long-term use may cause dependence, so you should discuss prolonged use of these medications with your physician.

Other medications frequently used to relieve back pain are antidepressants, which not only improve sleep and mood but are very good at providing pain relief.

Injections

Corticosteroid drugs, such as cortisone, are especially effective in decreasing inflammation. These drugs inhibit the production of prostaglandins and decrease white blood cells, immune-system blood cells, and the chemical products produced by these cells in the joints and tissues around them. If you have severe back pain that is not relieved by nonsteroidal anti-inflammatory drugs, your physician may suggest a corticosteroid injection into your spine. The medication is usually injected directly into points of special tenderness or pain in the muscles, into areas of compressed nerve roots, or near the facet joints. If you have fibrositis (see p.52) with pain affecting only specific areas, your physician may also inject a painkiller into the point where your pain originates (for example, a neck muscle). Sometimes a combination of a painkiller and a corticosteroid drug is the best treatment.

If treatment with corticosteroid medications seems effective, your physician may prescribe oral corticosteroids to control the condition. Often, this treatment is short-term; in a few conditions it is prescribed for longer periods. Some side effects, such as weight gain, excessive hair growth, fluid retention, and skin rash, may occur when taking corticosteroids for longer periods. It is important to remember that stopping this drug treatment must be done gradually. Do not stop taking these medications abruptly, and ask your physician about a safe way to reduce the dosage.

Some physicians inject chymopapain, an enzyme medication derived from the papaya plant, into a prolapsed disc. Some serious complications were linked to this procedure when it was first developed. One complication was a strong allergic reaction in people sensitive to papaya; an allergy skin test is now given before the procedure is performed. Few physicians perform this procedure today, mainly because of the risks and because its true benefits are questionable.

The enzyme used in chymopapain eats away the center of the disc, allowing it to shrink back to normal size, away from the nerve. The chymopapain thus eases your pain. The procedure, known as chemonucleolysis, does not work for all disc prolapse problems. Because the enzyme affects only the disc it is injected into, it cannot be used when the portion of the disc causing the pain has become detached from the rest of

43

the disc. The procedure should not be used if you also have spinal stenosis (see p.69) or have had a previous discectomy in the same place.

Braces, collars, and corsets

Braces, collars, and corsets help support and immobilize the spine as well as remind the wearer to stand and move properly.

A physician might suggest that you wear a collar after a neck injury or to support a weak disc in your cervical (neck) region. Braces and corsets support the trunk of the body and are often recommended after surgery on the back. All of these devices vary in size, flexibility, and materials used in constructing them. One type of brace, called a halo vest, keeps the head and neck straight inside a metal halo attached by rods to a kind of vest.

As a person recovers from surgery or as the back heals, most braces, corsets, and collars can be removed. Be sure to ask your physician how long you need to wear the device, and when. Your physician might want you to wear the device while playing a sport and during other times you feel your back may be unstable. Once you stop wearing the brace, your physician may recommend specific exercises to strengthen the muscles of your back and abdomen.

Traction

Traction is a treatment in which a pulling force is applied to the back to straighten the spine, to stretch joints and other tissues, and to immobilize the spine. Physicians use traction to treat cervical (neck) spinal injuries. For example, if fractured cervical vertebrae are out of alignment, your physician may use a head traction device to realign the bones. For head traction, tongs are placed on either side of the head and then connected to straps running over pulleys to weights that pull gently on the neck. The pulling effect of the device keeps the neck in proper alignment, which helps eliminate the pain while the vertebrae heal. (A halo vest—see previous page—may also be used to treat cervical vertebrae fractures.)

Traction of the cervical (neck) portion of the spine is also used to relieve compression of nerves in the neck and to reduce muscle spasm. However, spinal traction is no longer commonly used to treat lower back pain caused by a prolapsed disc.

Electrical stimulation

Electrical stimulation, formally called transcutaneous electrical nerve stimulation (TENS), is a treatment that applies tiny pulses of electricity to the skin to prevent the pain impulses from reaching the brain. The device is simple to use. However, most people receive no benefit from this treatment, and many physicians and scientists have questioned its effectiveness.

The equipment consists of a portable, battery-driven control unit with wires connected to electrodes that fasten to the body. With your physician's and physical therapist's help, you determine where to attach the electrodes at the sites of the pain and the strength and frequency of the electrical impulses. When you feel pain, you press a button, and tiny bursts of electricity stimulate the affected nerves. What you feel is a pricking or tingling sensation; it is not painful. You can wear the stimulator on a belt or carry it in your pocket.

The way in which this device works is not known. Yet the device does bring relief to some people with back pain, although the relief may not last indefinitely. Your physician can answer any questions you might have about this kind of therapy. **Warning:** Note that the electrical impulses of this device may interfere with cardiac pacemakers, so if you are wearing a pacemaker, never use electrical stimulation equipment.

Surgery

The majority of people who have back pain do not need surgery. Usually bed rest, drug therapy, and other treatments are effective. Occasionally, however, surgery becomes necessary when more conservative measures fail to work. On the other hand, prompt surgery may be recommended for conditions such as a spinal tumor or certain types of disc prolapse. (Disc prolapse occurs when the center of a disc ruptures through the cover and bulges out, pressing against a nerve root and causing back and/or leg pain; see p.54.)

Relieving pressure on a nerve caused by a disc prolapse is the most common reason for back surgery. Pressure on a nerve may be relieved by a laminectomy or laminotomy, in which part of the vertebra is removed to relieve pressure, and a discectomy, in which part of the ruptured disc is removed. For more detailed information, see Treatment for disc prolapse, p.57, and Types of disc prolapse surgery, p.58.

If several discs are affected, spinal fusion (see p.60) may be performed. Spinal fusion is a surgical procedure in which adjacent spinal vertebrae are fused together. This procedure is also performed to correct spinal instability caused by disease, spinal deformity, and severe fractures of the spine.

If surgery is a possibility, sit down with your physician and discuss any steps you may need to take in preparation (such as adjusting the dose of a medication that may interact with anesthesia), the surgical procedure, the expected benefits, and the possible complications. Learn what kind of rehabilitative care you will need after the procedure. Any kind of surgery is more likely to be successful if you know beforehand what to expect and what it will take to recover.

Risks

Any surgical procedure carries a risk. To begin with, there is a small risk of complications from anesthesia. There is also a risk of problems arising from other medical conditions such as heart or lung disease. And infection is always a possibility.

In thinking about back surgery, many people fear the danger of paralysis when the area around the spinal cord is manipulated. This is a small but real risk, especially with surgery in the cervical (neck) region. However, most surgeries (laminectomies with discectomies and spinal fusions are the most common) take place in the lumbar (lower back) region, to which the spinal cord does not extend. The spinal cord ends a few inches above the waist.

Another question is whether the operation will succeed. A high percentage of discectomies and fusions are successful in relieving pain. But success varies from person to person, depending on the severity of the condition, other back problems, and the individual's general health.

On the other hand, what is the risk of not undergoing the operation? Can the condition deteriorate to the point that you develop serious problems or even paralysis? Is the pain so unremitting and severe that it is both physically and emotionally debilitating? With a few exceptions, such as a tumor, severe disc prolapse, or an injury, back surgery is usually not an emergency. There is time to discuss all of these concerns with your physicians and to get a second opinion.

Pain clinics

The small number of people who continue to suffer pain despite treatment often can find the help they need to deal with their problem at a pain clinic. Most major medical centers have pain clinics.

At a pain clinic, teams of specialists help people learn to control pain, minimizing its effects on their lives without necessarily curing it. The emphasis is on a multidisciplinary approach, using the philosophy that the emotional as well as the physical aspects of chronic pain must be examined and managed.

If you visit a pain clinic, you will see a physician— an orthopedic surgeon, a neurologist, a neurosurgeon, or an anesthesiologist, depending on your condition. You might also see a psychiatrist (a physician who specializes in mental and emotional concerns), a psychologist, or a social worker.

The initial visit includes a medical history, tests, and a review of any medications you are taking. After interviews with various members of the team (some interviews also include your family members), the team meets to formulate an individualized plan of pain management. Many clinics encourage you to attend this meeting so that you can take control of the plan from the beginning. Often this initial meeting produces a contract between you (and maybe your spouse) and the treatment coordinator.

There are usually specific goals: working toward managing the pain, recognizing and compensating for the limitations that the pain imposes, gaining a perspective of the pain in relation to the other aspects of your life, and learning to accept an increase in pain without letting it once again take control.

To achieve these objectives, people attend educational sessions, relaxation training classes, and physical therapy. These sessions help you learn what provokes pain, how long you can expect it to last, and what you can do to alleviate or at least diminish it. Most of these sessions are group sessions, so that you can share your experiences with fellow pain sufferers and benefit from their support.

Decreasing tension and stress is also a major goal at pain clinics; that is why relaxation exercises are emphasized. But the specialists also use other techniques, sometimes including transcutaneous electrical nerve stimulation (TENS; see p.45), hypnosis, acupuncture, medications, and injections.

If you think a pain clinic might be helpful for you, discuss this option with your physician. Most clinics require a referral from a physician. Bear in mind, too, that some programs last for a few weeks while others require several months to complete.

If you hear about a pain clinic from a friend or neighbor, ask your physician if he or she recommends that clinic. Think twice if health care personnel at a clinic advise against a treatment recommended by your physician, especially if you are asked not to see other doctors as part of some new treatment program. And always ask your physician directly before discontinuing any medication or other treatment that he or she has prescribed for you.

BACK DISORDERS AND INJURIES

If you have a prolapsed disc (see p.54) that requires surgery, you are probably in great pain. If your back problem is common low back pain, your symptoms may be mild. This section describes the cause and symptoms of most common back disorders and injuries, so that you can have an idea of what to expect when you have back pain.

Muscle aches and pains

We are all susceptible to muscle cramps and spasms, particularly if our work or recreational activities demand strenuous physical exertion. But people who sit at a desk all day are vulnerable too, and it is wise for everyone to be aware of the symptoms of muscle problems.

Common low back pain

The lumbar (lower back) region is the most common site of back pain. This is because this portion of the back bears the heavy load of the weight of the upper body. This part of the spine is also subjected to a variety of bending, twisting, and side-to-side movements. It is not surprising that even a relatively insignificant abnormality can generate pain.

People between the ages of 30 and 60 are most commonly affected by lower back pain. This span coincides with most of a person's working life. Younger people usually have flexible spines, while age reduces spinal flexibility, protecting the spine by limiting its range of movement.

If your work or daily life involves heavy lifting and carrying, your risk of back pain increases. However, even people who sit for prolonged periods of time, especially in a cramped or bent-over position, place tremendous stress on their lower backs. For example, airline pilots and truck drivers are especially susceptible to low back pain.

Regardless of job conditions, if you are overweight, you risk being affected by back pain. Not only is your back carrying a heavier load, but the abdominal muscles that help support the spine may also be weakened. It is in your interest to lose weight to relieve your back.

What are the causes of low back pain? A very common cause is a strained muscle or ligament. Exercise, especially if it is vigorous or follows a long period of inactivity, or a sudden violent motion may cause a passing muscle spasm and a mild sprain to a ligament. If you feel a sudden sharp pain in your lower back, you have probably overextended the ligaments and muscles. This is a warning sign to stop what you are doing, particularly if you are lifting or stretching.

Other possible causes of low back pain include a prolapsed disc (see p.54) and facet joint displacement (see p.62). A prolapsed disc occurs when wear and tear along with pressure causes the soft center of the disc to protrude through the disc's outer layer. The protrusion presses on a nerve root emerging from the spine, causing pain. Facet joint displacement occurs when twisting movements of the spine cause two vertebrae to slip and lock out of place at a facet joint. Again, the displaced vertebrae may press on a nerve root.

Both prolapsed disc and facet joint displacement often cause spasms in the muscles overlying the affected joint. This increases the pain.

Physicians often cannot pinpoint the specific reason for back pain. This is especially true in those cases in which muscle and/or ligament strain is the culprit. Muscle and ligament strains or sprains usually cannot be detected by X rays and other tests. Even a prolapsed disc may be in its early stages and therefore not show on test results. When you have pain that cannot be verified by testing, this is what many physicians call nonspecific back pain. This does not mean that there is no cause or that the pain is not real. It simply means that your physician is unable to identify the cause of the pain.

In other cases, diagnostic tests do reveal the cause of low back pain. Muscle or ligament strain, a prolapsed disc, and facet joint displacement are considered to be mechanical causes of back pain; that is, none involves any underlying disease to be diagnosed.

Sometimes diseases cause back pain. A degenerative disease such as lumbar (lower back) osteoarthritis (see p.63) or ankylosing spondylitis (see p.66) may cause the pain. A stress fracture of a vertebra can generate pain. Also, a kidney infection can produce pain in the small of the back. Your physician will screen for these diseases if you have other symptoms or if it appears that more than a simple muscle strain is involved.

Common low back pain, including nonspecific pain, however, usually responds to treatment. Bed rest on a firm mattress, mild analgesic drugs, heat, and massage are often recommended as remedies for common low back pain. However, it is vital to be patient and recognize that healing the back takes time.

Fibrositis

Fibrositis, also called fibromyalgia or fibromyositis, is a painful inflammation of the connective tissue holding together the muscles and joints. Fibrositis can afflict any part of the back. It often occurs in the neck and shoulder areas, and the arms and legs as well. The aches and pains of fibrositis may be accompanied by areas of tenderness and painful nodules (lumps of tissue under the skin). A careful examination may also reveal muscles that are contracting continuously or in spasms.

The pain may begin gradually or suddenly and is aggravated by movement. Aching and stiffness appear in the areas affected by the nodules, which may cluster across the neck and shoulders but may also develop throughout the back and in the legs. Symptoms of depression sometimes accompany the condition, including anxiety, moodiness, loss of appetite, sleeplessness, loss of interest in life, or feelings of hopelessness and pessimism.

The cause of fibrositis is unknown, but it has been associated with some sleep disturbances and in a few cases may accompany other medical conditions. Your physician diagnoses it by ruling out other more serious diseases and can reassure you that fibrositis does not indicate a serious underlying disease. Most accompanying diseases are usually easy to treat.

Treatment of this condition is similar to that for low back pain: rest, heat, massage, and mild painkillers such as aspirin or ibuprofen. Antidepressant medications may also be prescribed if depression occurs. Sometimes the painful areas respond to an injection of an analgesic (pain-killing) drug. A program of gradually increasing aerobic exercise, better sleep and stress management, and low dosages of antidepressant medication often alleviate the symptoms. Tell your physician if you have heartburn at night or any other problems that might interfere with your sleep. Also, your physician may want to test your thyroid gland function.

Disorders and diseases

If you visit your physician because you are feeling pain in your back, he or she will most likely tell you that you are experiencing common low back pain. But in order to make this diagnosis or any diagnosis, your physician needs to examine you for signs of other diseases or disorders that can be causing your symptoms—if for no other reason than to rule them out. This section describes in detail some of the disorders that your physician needs to consider.

Prolapsed disc

Although this condition is popularly called a slipped disc, it is actually a ruptured, or herniated, disc. The discs between the spinal vertebrae are tightly bonded together and cannot "slip."

As discussed on p.7, between each two vertebrae is a pad of elastic cartilage called an intervertebral disc. Functioning as cushions between the vertebral bones, intervertebral discs have tough, fibrous outer covers and soft, elastic interiors. The elasticity of the disc gives the spine flexibility.

The aging process can have a harmful effect on the disc. After years of wear and tear, as well as pressure, on a disc, the outer cover becomes worn and may rupture. When this happens, the center, always under pressure, bulges out through the outer cover and presses against the nerve root. This pressure can, in turn, cause back and/or leg pain.

You may also feel the pain of a ruptured disc in other parts of your body, depending on which nerve root is compressed. If the ruptured disc presses on one of the roots of the sciatic nerve, you will feel pain down your buttock and perhaps numbness or weakness in the affected leg. A ruptured disc pressing on nerve roots in the neck may cause a shooting pain down the arm and numbness and muscle weakness in the hands and fingers. If the disc presses on the nerves in the cauda equina, which is the continuation of the spinal cord supplying the bladder and bowels, you may have trouble with either urinating or having bowel movements.

Much of the pain, numbness, or tingling will be aggravated by moving, coughing, or straining in any way.

The discs most likely to rupture are found in one of two places in the spine: the two lowermost discs in the lumbar (lower back) region and, slightly less likely, the lowermost discs in the cervical (neck) region. One of the reasons these two areas are more vulnerable is that they are mobile areas of the spine next to stiff sections; the flexible lumbar (lower back) region is next to the immobile sacrum, and the cervical discs are adjacent to the stiff thoracic (chest) region. Disc prolapses at other levels of the spine are uncommon.

Aging alone is not the only cause of disc problems. Although discs do degenerate and dry out as we get older, other factors may predispose a person to develop a prolapsed disc. For instance, sitting for long periods of time places more stress on the back and the discs than standing. (See How to select a comfortable chair, p.26.) Also, people who regularly do a great deal of lifting and/or twisting at work or during recreation are susceptible to disc problems.

A disc can also rupture suddenly with no warning from only a slight exertion. Lifting a toddler off the floor or groceries out of a car trunk can cause a rupture. However, this seemingly sudden rupture is usually the final result of a long process of degeneration that the person may not have realized was happening.

To diagnose the condition, your physician will want an exact description of when and where you feel the pain. During the examination, your physician will observe you while you are walking, sitting, standing, and bending. A person with a disc problem may stand more upright than usual and curve his or her back toward the side opposite the pain. Also, people with prolapsed discs usually feel significant leg pain.

PROLAPSED DISC

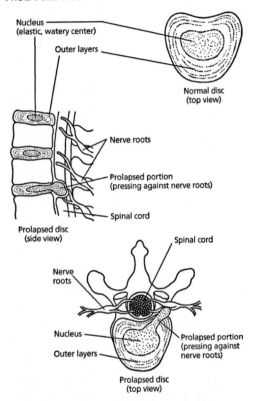

Nucleus (elastic, watery center)

Outer layers

Normal disc (top view)

Nerve roots

Prolapsed portion (pressing against nerve roots)

Spinal cord

Prolapsed disc (side view)

Spinal cord

Nerve roots

Nucleus

Prolapsed portion (pressing against nerve roots)

Outer layers

Prolapsed disc (top view)

The cross-sectional view from above shows that a disc (upper right) consists of an elastic, watery center (nucleus) surrounded by a tough, fibrous outer layer. If the outer layer becomes worn and thin, the center may prolapse, or rupture, through the outer layer and press against nerve roots, causing pain. The prolapsed portion is shown from the side (left) and from the top (bottom right).

The physician will then determine which nerve roots are irritated by placing your legs in various positions, by checking reflexes in the ankle and knee, by testing for sensation (using, for example, the light touch of a needle or hot or cold water on an arm or leg), and by testing muscle strength. If the tentative diagnosis is a disc prolapse, an X ray of the back may be taken to rule out other possible problems. Since regular X rays show bone better than they show the elastic disc, they often appear normal even when a disc is prolapsed. The tests used most commonly today are computed tomography (CT) scans and magnetic resonance imaging (MRI) scans, both of which show a cross section of the spine and the discs.

Treatment for disc prolapse

What is the treatment for a ruptured disc? Unless the rupture is severe, your physician will probably recommend the same nonsurgical treatment that is used with most back ailments. In the early stages this may consist of bed rest, anti-inflammatory drugs, pain medications, heat, and limitations in activity. Occasionally, a brace or corset is prescribed to immobilize the affected areas (see p.44). Injections of more powerful drugs may be given if the prolapsed disc does not respond to treatment. As the person becomes more mobile, physical therapy and learning methods of preventing back pain may help recovery. When the person returns to work depends on how much pain the person is experiencing.

If, however, the pressure from the disc is so great that it causes disabling muscle weakness, pain, or partial paralysis, surgery may be recommended. A discectomy may be performed to remove the protruding parts of the disc and relieve the compression on the nerve root. (See Types of disc prolapse surgery, on the next page.)

TYPES OF DISC PROLAPSE SURGERY

Disc prolapse surgery often involves more than one procedure, and the terms for these procedures can sound very similar. Here is a brief rundown on the surgical options for treating a prolapsed disc.

Most disc prolapse surgery begins with a laminotomy or a laminectomy, in which the surgeon removes either part or all of the lamina (the rear arch of the vertebra) in order to relieve pressure on the spinal cord caused by the prolapsed disc. If only part of the lamina needs to be shaved away to relieve the pressure, the procedure is called a laminotomy. If the entire lamina needs to be removed, the procedure is called a laminectomy.

In a discectomy, the protruding portion of the disc is removed. A laminectomy usually precedes a discectomy, because the laminectomy gives the surgeon access to the prolapsed disc.

If only a small portion of a disc needs to be removed, your surgeon may be able to perform a microdiscectomy. In this procedure, a less invasive form of discectomy (the lamina remains intact), the surgeon makes a small incision and uses very small surgical instruments with the aid of an operating microscope or other magnifying device.

After general anesthesia is administered for the discectomy (making the patient unconscious), the patient is turned facedown on his or her stomach. The site of the prolapsed disc is checked ahead of time using a CT (computed tomography) or MRI (magnetic resonance imaging) scan. An incision is made in the back, and muscles are drawn back to expose the underlying bony spine, and specifically the lamina (the rear arch of a vertebra). Cutting instruments are then commonly used to shave or remove part or all of the lamina in order to safely gain access to the spine. The flaval ligament, which envelops the spinal canal, is partially

TYPES OF DISC PROLAPSE SURGERY

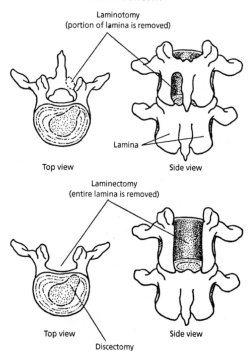

Laminotomy
(portion of lamina is removed)

Lamina

Top view

Side view

Laminectomy
(entire lamina is removed)

Top view

Side view

Discectomy
(prolapsed portion of disc is removed)

removed to expose the nerve root and the underlying herniated disc. Many surgeons use a magnifying device, such as a set of loupes (magnifying glasses), in performing discectomies.

Pulling the nerve root aside, the surgeon removes the ruptured disc material and any other loose disc material from the site. After making certain that the nerve is no longer being compressed, the surgeon closes the incision. You are allowed to get out of bed the following day, and full recovery generally occurs over a few weeks to a few months. You are usually advised to resume daily activities gradually, including return to work.

If only a small amount of tissue needs to be removed, your disc prolapse may be treated with an operation called a microdiscectomy. Making a small incision into the skin and the tissues over the disc, the surgeon uses an operating microscope or other magnifying device and special instruments to remove the protruding parts of the disc; the lamina may not need to be removed. The surgery poses fewer risks of complications, leaves only a small scar, and requires only a few days' stay in a hospital.

Depending on the underlying condition, the surgeon may recommend a spinal fusion, in which two or more adjacent vertebrae are fused together. Bone grafts taken from the person's pelvic bone are used as a bridge over which new permanent bone will grow, knitting the vertebrae together solidly.

After the administration of a general anesthetic, the surgeon makes an incision and gains access under the muscles to the bony parts of the spine. The vertebrae are prepared for fusion by removing thin slivers of bone from their sides. Bone for grafting is taken from the pelvic bone and placed on the prepared sides of the vertebrae. When the muscles slide back into place, they hold the grafts in position. To increase the chances of the fusion healing properly, sometimes a metal fixation device is used to provide additional support. The surgeon closes the incision, leaving a drain in place to prevent fluid buildup.

After a spinal fusion, you may be immediately fitted with a brace for back support. After several months, if X rays show that the bones are fusing together satisfactorily, the brace is removed.

The spinal fusion operation is also used for spinal instability, caused by a vertebra slipping forward, for unstable fractures of the spine, or for spinal deformities such as scoliosis.

In older people, bony growths on the vertebrae as a result of osteoarthritis (see p.63) may eventually compress the nerve root or cauda equina (see p.8), causing pain, numbness, difficulty walking, and loss of nerve function. This condition is known as spinal stenosis (see p.69). If symptoms do not clear up with nonsurgical measures (see Types of treatment, p.38), surgery may be required. The surgical approach is similar to that in a discectomy, except that the obstructing bone is removed instead of a portion of a disc. A spinal fusion with or without a fixation device may be necessary, depending on the quantity of bone removed.

Sciatica

Sciatica is pain that travels along the path of the sciatic nerves. Formed by the combination of several nerves that emerge from the lower part of the spine, the sciatic nerves, one on each side, travel down the buttocks and the back of the thigh to the knee. From there the nerves branch into other nerves. Therefore, sciatic pain begins in the lower back and moves into the hip, buttocks, and the back of the thigh.

The most common cause of sciatica is a prolapsed disc in a location such that its bulging contents press against the sciatic nerve roots. Thus, the treatment options are the same as those for a prolapsed disc: rest, painkillers, heat, traction, or braces. If the sciatica becomes debilitating, however, surgery may be necessary.

It is important to note that sciatica can be a symptom of other problems, including tumors, infections, injuries, and arthritis. Your physician will want to rule out these possibilities or to treat a disorder or condition if one exists.

Facet joint displacement

Another common cause of sudden back pain is a facet joint displacement, which occurs when a twisting movement of the spine causes two vertebrae to slip and lock out of place at a facet joint.

Normally, a vertebra does not slip. However, a flaw or a crack can allow the rear portion of the vertebra with its facet joints to detach from the front part. The vertebra can then slip out of alignment with the other bones in the spine. Some physicians think that the flaw occurs because of a hereditary weakness worsened by long-term wear and tear.

Many people can control the pain of facet joint displacement with the same nonsurgical routines suggested for prolapsed disc, including corsets or braces to support the spine. A small number of people, however, may need surgery to correct the condition before it causes more degeneration and displacement in the spine. In those cases, spinal fusion surgery is performed to bring the displaced vertebra into alignment with the other vertebrae.

Other possible spinal conditions

As described on p.54, when examining you to determine the cause of your back pain, your physician makes an effort to rule out as many diseases as possible. Some of these diseases are profiled here.

Arthritis

Arthritis means inflammation of the joints. Characterized by joint pain, swelling, and stiffness, arthritis is one of the leading causes of disability. Although the many kinds of arthritis share common symptoms, they differ in their causes, symptoms, and resulting damage. The three most common forms affecting the back are osteoarthritis, rheumatoid arthritis, and ankylosing spondylitis. Rheumatoid arthritis and ankylosing spondylitis are considered forms of inflammatory arthritis, because they involve inflammation (swelling) of the membranes surrounding the joints. Osteoarthritis is considered noninflammatory, because it involves degeneration of the cartilage tissue in the joint.

OSTEOARTHRITIS

The most common form of arthritis is osteoarthritis, also called degenerative arthritis. It can result from general wearing away of the cartilage, the elastic tissue that cushions the joints and prevents the bones from actually touching, or it can be caused by an injury to the cartilage. It affects almost everyone over the age of 60, particularly women.

As cartilage breaks down, its surfaces become rough and gradually thinner as they grind against each other. Small pieces of cartilage break off and irritate the synovial membrane, the thin lining that produces lubricating fluid in the interior of the joint. The result is an inflamed, painful membrane that may also contribute to limited movement of the joint. Eventually with osteoarthritis, most of the cartilage is worn away so that bone grates against bone.

The symptoms of osteoarthritis are pain, swelling, tenderness, stiffness, or redness in one or more joints. Often the stiffness is worse in the morning and improves as you move about during the day. Sometimes, the pain increases toward the end of the day.

The best results are achieved with a program of drug therapy, rest, and exercise. Because arthritic joints are often the cause of pain in the weight-bearing portion of the back, the nonsurgical treatment (see Types of treatment, p.38) for relieving low back pain is usually recommended. Nonsteroidal anti-inflammatory drugs

(NSAIDs), such as aspirin, and heat therapy are often quite effective. Reducing strain on your joints is very important; maintaining your proper weight and avoiding heavy lifting can slow down joint irritation.

It is important also to establish a regular schedule of moderate exercise to maintain and improve the flexibility of your joints. Talk with your physician about an exercise program that will help your joints without placing any unnecessary strain on them.

In very severe cases of osteoarthritis, the joint may be immobilized or replaced.

RHEUMATOID ARTHRITIS

Rheumatoid arthritis is the most serious form of inflammatory arthritis. The cause is not known, although it is thought that some people inherit characteristics that can increase their susceptibility. The events that trigger rheumatoid arthritis are also not known. (Related types of inflammatory arthritis are sometimes triggered by an isolated event, such as an infection.) Once triggered, rheumatoid arthritis acts like an autoimmune condition in which the body attacks its own tissues. Rheumatoid arthritis usually affects mainly the cervical (neck) area of the spine along with other joints in the arms and legs. Other types of inflammatory arthritis affect the lower back.

In rheumatoid arthritis, the synovial membrane that lines the tough fibrous layers surrounding a joint becomes inflamed. As the inflammation continues, it destroys the cartilage between the bones. Eventually, the damaged cartilage is replaced by scar tissue, making the joint rigid and altering its shape.

Early in an attack the person feels tired and ill and then experiences joint pain and stiffness. The affected joints become swollen, warm, red, and stiff. Also, spreading inflammation may cause weakness in the ligaments and muscles around the joints. Most commonly rheumatoid arthritis causes pain and symptoms of nerve compression. As the disease progresses, it affects more and more joints, which do not work well and often become deformed.

While rheumatoid arthritis does not usually begin in the spine, it can spread to that area. The disease most commonly attacks the upper neck, damaging the facet joints in the uppermost cervical (neck) vertebrae. This form of arthritis can also damage discs and parts of nearby vertebrae. You may need to exercise precautions suggested by your physician, if you have rheumatoid arthritis of the cervical (neck) spine.

Treatment for rheumatoid arthritis is aimed primarily at relieving symptoms, preventing joints from becoming deformed, and preserving the motion of joints. The reliable standbys of rest, nonsteroidal anti-inflammatory drugs (NSAIDs) to relieve pain and inflammation, and exercise to maintain mobility are the cornerstones of treating this disease. If there are signs the disease is persisting despite treatment, the physician may prescribe an antirheumatic drug, such as sulfasalazine, penicillamine, or chloroquine (which is also used to treat malaria), to slow its progress. Compounds with gold are also used to treat rheumatoid and other forms of arthritis.

Because rheumatoid arthritis acts like a disorder of the body's immune system, drugs that suppress the immune system, such as corticosteroid drugs, are sometimes used in treatment. Methotrexate, an anticancer drug, is also used to treat rheumatoid arthritis.

Eventually, surgery may be necessary to stabilize or repair ligaments, to release joint contractures (deformities caused by scar tissue) or tendons entrapped by joint inflammation or scar tissue, or to remove inflamed synovial membranes from the joints. At this point, depending on how deformed and immobile the joint is, replacing the joint with an artificial joint may be recommended. This is reserved for advanced cases but can often relieve pain and allow you to move those joints again.

ANKYLOSING SPONDYLITIS

Ankylosing spondylitis is also a serious inflammatory joint disease. Ankylosing means fusing, and spondylitis means inflammation of the vertebrae. Beginning usually before the age of 30, this condition is often dismissed as a strained back. In reality, the inflammation starts at the base of the spine in the sacroiliac (sacrum/pelvis) joint and moves up the spine, sometimes as far as the cervical spine, destroying the cartilage in the discs and replacing it with scar tissue that eventually turns to bone. The outcome may be that the vertebrae become fused together in a solid, rigid rod, which may leave your head permanently bent down to your chest and leave you more susceptible to spinal fractures. Sometimes the disease also fuses the ends of the ribs, hindering breathing, and attacks the hips and shoulders.

The cause of this disease is not known, but, as in rheumatoid arthritis, there seems to be a genetic connection. Also as in rheumatoid arthritis, there may be a defect in the immune system.

Early symptoms are pain and stiffness in the back. Using abdominal muscles to breathe rather than expanding the rib cage is another clue. But a telltale sign of ankylosing spondylitis is that, unlike other types of back pain, bed rest aggravates the pain of this disease rather than relieving it.

If diagnosed and treated early, the person is able to live a nearly normal life. Medications, including painkillers and anti-inflammatory drugs, are the first treatment. Therapists teach people with this condition techniques for maintaining as erect a posture as possible, both during the day and at night. Therapy also involves deep breathing exercises and other special exercises to keep the spine and related joints flexible, or at least in a good posture if the bones become fused.

Osteoporosis and osteomalacia

These two bone disorders are related to hormonal and/or nutritional imbalances. Bones affected by osteoporosis are weak, less dense, and easily fractured. There is a reduction in bone tissue, which in turn leads to a reduction in the deposits of calcium, which is vital to building and maintaining strong bones. As osteoporosis advances, there are simply not enough areas in the body's bony framework to accept calcium deposits to maintain strong bones.

Osteomalacia, on the other hand, does not reduce the density of the bones. In this condition, your bones do not thin so much as soften. The softening occurs because of a loss of calcium and phosphorus, minerals necessary for strong bones. The mineral loss is usually due to a deficiency of vitamin D. (Rickets, a similar disorder, affects children.)

As part of the process in which bone is broken down and then reformed, a good supply of calcium and phosphorus is necessary. Vitamin D is essential for the absorption of calcium from the intestines and for the reduction of phosphorus elimination through the kidneys. Any interference with this vital balance leads to abnormally low levels of calcium and phosphorus in the blood, and subsequent loss of these minerals from the bones.

What causes a vitamin D deficiency? There are three main factors—inadequate intake in your diet, lack of exposure to sunlight, or poor absorption of the vitamin from the intestines. A kidney disorder may also contribute to the deficiency.

Symptoms of osteomalacia include bone pain and tenderness, often in the neck, ribs, hips, and legs. Difficulty walking and sleeplessness may be brought about by pain. Low levels of calcium in the blood can also cause painful muscle spasms. X-ray tests may show weakened ribbonlike areas in bone and vertebrae that are concave (curved inward) on their upper and lower surfaces.

Treatment almost always improves the condition. Changing your diet is relatively easy; look for foods that are rich in vitamin D, such as dairy products (low-fat or nonfat items are preferable) or oily fish, and for products fortified with vitamin D. If a kidney problem or a fat absorption malfunction in the intestine prevents you from absorbing enough vitamin D (a fat-soluble vitamin), your physician will treat these underlying conditions. Sunlight forms vitamin D in your skin naturally. If you have little or no exposure to the sun because you are housebound or live in a smoggy area, you can take vitamin D supplements.

Osteoporosis is also treated with calcium and vitamin D intake, to avoid further bone loss. Osteoporosis, however, is best avoided by prevention. Adequate intake of calcium and vitamin D and weight-bearing exercise are all preventive measures that should be continued throughout life. The prevention aspect of this disease cannot be stated too strongly; you can prevent or slow bone loss, but you cannot replace bone already lost.

For people who have lost significant amounts of bone, as shown by increased fractures, loss of height from compression fractures of the vertebrae, or aches and pains, research continues to seek treatments. In addition to hormone replacement therapy, several other treatments are under investigation. Sodium fluoride stimulates the formation of new bone, but the new material may be weak. The drug etidronate is capable of increasing bone density, but physicians are still studying its place in osteoporosis treatment. The thyroid hormone calcitonin is also being studied, but it has undesirable side effects. Again, the best therapy is still prevention.

Spinal stenosis

This condition is a narrowing in the spine. Stenosis means narrowing, and in the spine the problem can occur in the central spinal canal or in the openings at the sides of the vertebrae through which the nerve roots pass. These narrowed passageways can cause pressure and pain in the back.

The condition can be congenital—that is, present from birth—or due to injury or to facet joint displacement (see p.62). The most common cause of spinal stenosis, however, is degenerative arthritis, also called osteoarthritis, which produces bony thickening of the edges of the vertebrae.

The symptoms depend on the location of the narrowing. If the stenosis occurs in the central spinal column, you will feel low back pain with numbness, tingling, and cramps in the legs. Walking worsens the symptoms, and you may be forced to stop to rest. One interesting aspect is that the dimension of the spinal canal is larger when the spine is bent forward. Therefore, you may find walking painful, but bicycling with your body bent over the handlebars may cause no pain at all.

When the openings in the sides of the vertebrae are narrowed, this may cause pressure on the nerve roots. For example, stenosis in the neck can produce tingling and numbness in the arms. In the lumbar (lower back) region, narrowing can cause the shooting pain of sciatica (see p.61). The type and location of symptoms helps pinpoint the site of the narrowing.

Sophisticated tests such as CT (computed tomography) or MRI (magnetic resonance imaging) scans are also necessary to locate the exact cause of the problems. This is important because treatment often requires surgery to enlarge the narrowed passageways.

Scoliosis

Scoliosis is a condition in which the spine develops a sideways curve, usually in the lower back or chest portions of the spine. Scoliosis usually begins in childhood but may not be noticeable until adolescence. The curvature can be caused by bone or muscle abnormalities, but more often there is no obvious cause. Although the deformity usually does not cause great pain, scoliosis gets worse over time if not treated and eventually may cause pain and, in severe cases, difficulty breathing. For milder cases, a metal brace or plaster cast may be used to keep the spine straight. More severe deformities can be treated with surgery, by spinal fusion (see p.60), or by inserting metal rods next to the spine.

Cancer affecting the spine

Bone cancer in the spine is uncommon. Of the tumors or growths that do affect the spine, most originate elsewhere in the body and spread to the spine. A tumor on the spine may eventually compress nerves, causing symptoms similar to those of a prolapsed disc (see p.54). Benign (noncancerous) tumors, such as those called meningiomas or neurofibromas, sometimes originate in the tissues in the spine, but are rare. Most other spinal tumors are malignant (cancerous). Spinal tumors can be removed through surgery; however, the earlier the growth is detected, the better the chances are for successful removal and recovery.

Cancer in the abdomen (stomach area) and pelvic organs can produce back pain, sometimes as the first symptom, although this is rare. When you see a physician about persistent back pain, he or she will conduct tests to rule out cancer and other serious diseases.

Injuries

Anyone who suffers an injury to the back needs careful and special attention. Not only are the vertebrae, muscles, ligaments, and other structures of the back subject to harm, but also there is a grave danger of damage to the spinal cord. A compressed or severed spinal cord and injury to the spinal nerves can cause paralysis (loss of movement and feeling) below the site of the injury all the way to the toes.

For example, a spinal cord cut at the neck can cause death instantly or turn the person into a quadriplegic (a person without the ability to move or to feel anything in the arms, trunk, or legs). If the cord is cut near the waist, the person can become a paraplegic, unable to move or feel anything in the lower trunk or the legs.

Warning: It is critical *not* to move a person suspected to have a back or neck injury without medical assistance. In fact, a good rule of thumb is to *always assume spinal injury in an accident.* Any movement or twisting of a person with such an injury can shift broken bone debris or misaligned back components and jeopardize the spinal cord and nerves.

The only exception to this rule is if the victim's life is in danger. Move the victim *only* if there is life-threatening danger, such as a fire, explosion, drowning, cave-in, or approaching traffic. If you are forced to move the person, immobilize his or her neck and back. Place a wide board under the head, neck, and back, keeping them aligned. Support the sides of the head and neck with rolled-up blankets, clothes, or pieces of rock or wood. When you move the victim, keep the neck and back straight, support them, and do not let the head, neck, or back fall or twist to the side.

Cervical (neck) spine injury

Cervical (neck) injuries often cause damage to the spinal cord and nerves. Severe injuries can cause total paralysis; a less severe injury can result in partial paralysis and loss of sensation. Most critical of all, injuries involving the top four cervical vertebrae can be instantly fatal or, if not fatal, damaging to the nerves that control breathing. In these cases, artificial ventilation (machine breathing) may become vital.

Diagnosis and treatment of cervical spinal injuries are crucial to recovery. The examination and tests must be done in such a way that the neck and, in some cases, the back remain immobilized until the extent of the injuries can be determined.

Traction is often used to treat fractured cervical vertebrae that are misaligned. The therapist may securely place on each side of the head a device with weights attached to pull gently on the neck. Traction realigns the vertebrae and allows them to heal. Or, in place of traction, a halo vest (see p.44) may be used to stabilize the vertebrae.

If injuries cause instability in the cervical spine, an operation to fuse the vertebrae at the site of the injury may be necessary. After surgery the patient may have to wear a soft foam cervical collar or a brace for a few months to support the neck while it heals.

Cervical (neck) strain or sprain

A less serious cervical (neck) injury occurs when the muscles, discs, and joints of the neck are strained or sprained because the neck is unnaturally forced forward or backward. For example, if someone hits your car from behind, your head is suddenly thrown backward and your neck bent farther than normal (this is sometimes called "whiplash"). Using a properly adjusted car headrest and wearing a seat and shoulder belt can help make this type of injury less severe.

A flexing injury occurs if your car is hit head-on and your neck is forced forward or flexed. Your chin will strike your chest, which stops the forward movement of your head.

Both of these injuries may cause neck pain and stiffness accompanied by aching across the shoulders and down the arms. However, symptoms may not develop until 6 to 12 hours after the incident. After checking for a more serious injury, your physician will probably suggest taking painkilling drugs (such as aspirin or ibuprofen, or acetaminophen with codeine for more severe pain) and wearing a soft foam neck collar for a few days. Physical therapy may be necessary if symptoms persist.

Spinal injury—crush and burst fracture

Often a serious fall can fracture a vertebra. A crush fracture results from pressure on the spine when it is bent or flexed; the front part of the vertebra collapses. People with osteoporosis can suffer this kind of vertebral fracture even after minor falls. A crush fracture seldom causes damage to the spinal cord and nerves.

A more serious fracture, a burst fracture, occurs when a force presses on the spine when it is straight. This kind of fracture can cause damage to the nerves.

Both fractures cause pain in the vicinity of the vertebrae. Bed rest and exercises to maintain mobility are usually recommended. Some people may need a spinal brace for a few weeks, a few months, or longer.

Burst fractures may require a long period of recuperation. In addition, some of these injuries require surgery to stabilize the spine. Very severe fractures are often treated in the same way as cervical spine injuries, with traction and surgery.

Infection

Infection of the spine by bacteria is not common, but such an infection can become a very serious problem, especially if it is not diagnosed and treated early. Bacteria can find their way into the spine during spinal surgery or injections, from nearby infections, or through the bloodstream. Osteomyelitis, an infection of bone and bone marrow, is caused mainly by staphylococcus bacteria. In adults, the bacteria often attack the vertebrae and the pelvis. Once in the spine, the bacteria cause pain; muscle spasm; tender bones, muscle, and skin; and fever. The disc tissue may become infected as well. If untreated, the disease can become chronic and very difficult to cure. Tuberculosis can also attack the spine, but this is now rare.

Occasionally a spinal infection causes an abscess to form in the space in the spinal canal next to the spinal cord called the epidural space. An epidural abscess is a medical emergency and requires prompt treatment. Symptoms include increasingly severe pain in the spine, increasing feelings of numbness or weakness, and fever. If you experience these symptoms, get medical help immediately.

CONCLUSION

Much of this book consists of descriptions of all the illnesses and injuries that may affect your back, mildly or severely. Taking a little time for preventive back care today usually pays off handsomely in the future. To begin, control your weight and make sure you get enough calcium to ward off osteoporosis. Start a regular exercise program that includes exercises to keep your back muscles strong and flexible and your joints limber (see p.31). Review the basics of good posture (see p.22) and practice them, so that they become second nature to you. There is a right way and a wrong way to bend and lift; be sure you know the right way (see p.28).

If your back begins to hurt, pay attention to your symptoms (see p.36) and consult your physician. An added benefit of taking steps to care for your back is that the rest of your body may benefit, too.

GLOSSARY

Analgesic drug   A pain reliever.

Ankylosing spondylitis   Inflammatory disease that fuses together the vertebrae of the back.

Atlas   The first spinal vertebra, which supports the skull.

Axis   The second spinal vertebra, which, in conjunction with the atlas, allows movement of the head.

Burst fracture   Broken vertebrae caused by direct pressure against a straight spine.

Cauda equina (horse's tail)   Individual nerve fibers that continue from the end of the spinal cord down the spinal canal in strands that resemble a horse's tail.

Cervical   Pertaining to the neck region of the spine.

Coccyx   Final four fused vertebrae in the spinal column.

Compression fracture   Broken vertebrae caused by vertebrae collapsing under their own weight, compressing the spine.

Corticosteroid   Steroidal drug that decreases inflammation and pain.

Crush fracture   Broken vertebrae resulting from pressure on the spine when it is bent or flexed, collapsing the front part of the vertebrae.

Disc   Pad of cartilage tissue between two vertebrae that acts as a cushion and shock absorber for the spine; also called intervertebral disc.

Discectomy   Surgical procedure to remove the protruding part of a prolapsed disc to eliminate pressure on a nerve root. See also Microdiscectomy.

Endorphins   Pain-relieving substances that occur naturally in the brain.

Erector spinae Group of back muscles running the entire length of the spine that supports and manipulates the spine.

Exercise, weight-bearing See Weight-bearing exercise.

Facet joint The joint between two vertebrae that allows movement of the spine and prevents forward slippage.

Facet joint displacement Condition in which two or more vertebrae slip and lock out of place at a facet joint.

Fibrositis Painful inflammation of the connective tissue components of the muscles and joints; also called fibromyalgia or fibromyositis.

Halo vest An apparatus used to stabilize vertebrae in treating fractures of the neck.

Hormones Chemicals responsible for controlling a wide range of body functions; produced by different glands and organs.

Hormone replacement therapy Hormones given as medication to replace hormones missing from the body or to increase low levels of hormones. Estrogen replacement therapy, in which estrogen hormones alone are given to treat the symptoms of menopause and osteoporosis, is a form of hormone replacement therapy.

Laminectomy Procedure in which the rear arch of the vertebra (the lamina) is removed to relieve pressure on a nerve root. See also Laminotomy.

Laminotomy Procedure in which only part of the lamina bone is removed from a vertebra to relieve pressure on a nerve root. See also Laminectomy.

Ligament Tough band of connective tissue connecting one bone to another.

Lumbar Pertaining to the lower back region of the spine.

Microdiscectomy Procedure using microsurgical techniques to remove the protruding part of a prolapsed disc to eliminate pressure on a nerve root.

Nerve root Any of the nerve bundles that branch off the spinal cord.

Nonspecific back pain Pain for which no cause has yet been found.

Nonsteroidal anti-inflammatory drug (NSAID) A drug that fights pain and inflammation but is not a corticosteroid—examples: aspirin, ibuprofen.

Osteoarthritis A condition in which the cartilage in the joints wears away, causing irritation and painful, swollen joints.

Osteomalacia Softening of the bones due to a vitamin D deficiency.

Osteoporosis A condition in which the bones lose mass and become weak and easily fractured; insufficient calcium intake and lack of the female sex hormone estrogen contribute to the disease.

Osteosarcoma The most common bone cancer that starts in the bones.

Paralysis Complete or partial loss of sensation and movement.

Process A projection of the vertebra that serves as an attachment site for the back muscles.

Prolapsed disc A condition in which the center of an intervertebral disc ruptures and protrudes through the outer layer or cover, pressing on a nerve root and causing pain.

Prostaglandins Substances in the body that perform hormonelike actions including triggering pain and inflammation.

Recommended dietary allowance (RDA) Recommended levels of essential nutrients to be included in a healthy diet, as determined by the National Research Council.

Rheumatoid arthritis Chronic inflammatory joint disease.

Sacrum The five fused vertebrae directly above the coccyx.

Sciatic nerve One of a pair of the largest nerves in the body, which form in the lower back and travel through the hip region down the back of the thigh.

Sciatica Pain that travels the pathway of the sciatic nerve.

Scoliosis An abnormality of the back in which the spine is curved to one side of the normally vertical line.

Spinal cord A cylinder of nerve tissue that runs directly from the brain down the central canal in the spine.

Spinal fusion Surgical procedure that welds adjacent vertebrae together.

Spinal stenosis Narrowing in the spinal column, involving either or both the spinal canal or the nerve root openings.

Spinous process The projection that points backward from the vertebrae. See Process.

Swayback Exaggerated inward curvature of the spine.

Synovial membrane The thin membrane that lines the inside of the fibrous outer covering of a movable joint.

Thoracic Pertaining to the chest region of the spine.

Traction A pulling force applied to the body to straighten or stretch tissues.

Transcutaneous electrical nerve stimulation (TENS) An unproven method of treatment involving application of tiny electrical pulses to the skin to prevent pain impulses from reaching the brain.

Transverse processes Side projections of vertebrae that serve as attachment sites for the back muscles.

Vertebra   A bone in the spinal column.

Weight-bearing exercise   Physical activity that puts pressure or weight on bones; needed to maintain bone strength and health.

INDEX

INDEX

NOTES

NOTES